WOMEN AND CANCER
HALA GOMA, MD,
PROFESSOR OF ANESTHESIA CAIRO UNIVERSITY

Table of contents

Introduction

One of the top women diseases is cancer, the most cancers affect women are cancer breast, lung, and colorectal cancer. The predisposing causes of cancer are tobacco, obesity, radiation, genetic factor play an important cause for these cancers. Cancer may be present in certain families. Preoperative preparation is very important for these patient, anesthetist must take many factors in consideration during preoperative evaluation .effect of chemotherapy on different body system, and chemotherapy may produce cardio toxic, pulmonary, hepato-renal, and hematological effects. Proper evaluation for ischemic heart disease, congestive heart failure, diabetes, and chronic renal failure .This book discus the risk factors and the preoperative preparation for cancer patient.

Cancer common in women

- **Breast cancer** is the leading cancer for women in the US.
- **Lung cancer** is the second most common form of cancer
- **Colorectal cancer** is third among white women. The number 2 and 3 cancers are reversed among black and Asian/Pacific Island women.
- For all women, the fourth leading cancer is cancer of the **uterus**.

Possible causes of cancer

Environmental factors.

- Common environmental factors that contribute to cancer death include
- Tobacco (25–30%), diet and obesity (30–35%),
- Infections (15–20%),
- Radiation (both ionizing and non-ionizing, up to 10%),
- stress,
- lack of physical,
- environmental pollutants
- inherited genetics
- The remaining 5–10% are due.
- Lifestyle, economic and behavioral factors, and not merely pollution.

General symptoms

- unintentional weight loss,
- **fever**,
- being excessively tired,
- changes to the skin **Hodgkin disease**,
- **leukemias**, and liver or **kidney** can cause a persistent **fever of unknown origin**

- most common places for metastases to occur are the **lungs**, **liver**, **brain**, and the bone

Cancer and anesthesia

Preoperative Evaluation

- Already systemic diseases ad hypertension , diabetes, ischemic heart diseases
- General complications of cancer, as anemia, loss of weight
- Specific tumor complications, as electrolytes imbalance due to vomiting
- Metastasis in the lung, liver ,bone
- Chemotherapy and radiation systemic effects

Preoperative Preparation

- Electrolyte abnormalities are common in patients with abdominal pain or vomiting, thus consider a preoperative chem.
- Blood products available + Ranger / rapid infuser.
- Cefoxitin (do not give SQ heparin (5000 U) until AFTER the epidural, if placed).

Most common causes of death of cancer patients

Sepsis, hemorrhage, and cardiovascular events Induction/Airway: if the tumor is obstructive, consider RSI.

Intraoperative management

- Lines and Monitors:
- two large-bore IVs,
- Arterial line (frequent labs, esp. glucose).
- Central line.
- general +/- epidural (T6-8, inferior angle of scapula is approximately T7

Epidural anesthesia

- opiate-enhanced epidural is used, consider a lipophilic drug (ex.fentanyl),
- morphine will potentially spread rostrally,
- Potentially causing mental status changes and respiratory depression.
- Consider 0.5%bupivacaine intraoperatively, followed by 0.125% – 0.25% post-operatively.

- In patients for whom an epidural is not possible, consider ketamine at 0.2 mg/kg/hr after a 0.5 mg/kg bolus, as well as gabapentin 600-1200 mg PO.

Intraoperative Goals and Events:
- Placement of nasogastric tube (will be used post-operatively).
- WARM maintenance fluids at 6-10 cc/kg/hr.

Postoperative management
- Emergence: depends on fluid shifts and cardiopulmonary status. May remain intubated.
- ICU admission.
- Epidural-trained ward if epidural in place.

Cancer patients undergo chemotherapy before being subjected for surgery. Such patients pose some serious interactions and complications during the anesthetic management.

Common complications associated with cancer chemotherapy agents

System toxicity	Chemotherapeutic agents
Cardiac toxicity	Busulphan, cisplatin, cyclophosphamide, daunorubucin, 5-fluorouracil
Pulmonary toxicity	Methotrexate, bleomycin, busulphan, cyclophosphamide, cytarabine, carmustine
Renal toxicity	Methotrexate, L-asparginase, carboplatin,

System toxicity	Chemotherapeutic agents
	ifosfamide, mitomycin-C
Hepatic toxicity	Actinomycin D, methotrexate, androgens, L-asparginase, busulphan, cisplatinum, azathiopine
CNS toxicity	Methotrexate, cisplatin, interferon, hydroxyurea, procarbazine, vincristine
SIADH secretion	Cyclophosphamide, vincristine

The most common toxicities to chemotherapeutic agents

- Cardiac,
- Pulmonary,
- Hematologic,
- Bone marrow
- Gastrointestinal effects.
- Coagulopathies, thrombocytopenia,
- anemia with ulceration and bleeding of the gastrointestinal tract

Cardiovascular effects and complications following chemotherapy

Anthracyclines; i.e. doxorubicin (adriamycin), daunorubicin, and epirubicinare the commonest agents implicated in the development of cardiac toxicity after cancer chemotherapy.

Three types depending on their appearance in relation to timing of therapy,

Anthracycline agents may impair myocardial contractility.

Risk factors for development of anthracycline cardiotoxicity:

1. high dose radiation to the mediastinum
2. concurrent cyclophosphamide therapy
3. extremes of age,
4. prior ischemic heart disease,
5. hypertension,
6. Valvular heart disease and liver diseases.
7. Cumulative dose in the range of 300-450 mg/m2 is about 1-10%, while doses higher than this invites a risk of>30%.

Pathogenesis of anthracycline cardio toxicity:

- The anthracycline antibiotics react with cytochrome P-450 reductase in the presence of reduced nicotinamide adenine dinucleotide phosphate to form semi Quinone radical intermediates, which in turn can react with oxygen to form superoxide anion radicals.

- These can generate both hydrogen peroxide and hydroxyl radicals, which are highly destructive to cells thus causing myofibrillarlysis, cytoplasmic vacuolization, and degeneration of nuclei and mitochondria in the myocytes. Severe myocyte damage results in decreased myocardial contractility and CHF.

Investigations for the detection of anthracycline cardiotoxicity:

- Radionucleide angiocardiography. The

- Left ventricular ejection fraction (LVEF). A decrease in LVEF to less than 45% is considered to indicate anthracycline-induced cardio toxicity. 2-Dechocardiography is a non-invasive method of cardiac valuation.
- Diastolic dysfunction on echocardiogram may represent an earlier manifestation of anthracycline toxicity.
- The newer noninvasive methods to know the actual myocardial damage are by using imaging with monoclonal indium–111–antimyosin antibodies.
- These antibodies bind to the exposed myosin in the necrosed myocardial cells.
- A diffuse uptake on imaging indicates a generalized process such as anthracycline cardiomyopathy; a focal uptake will suggest local pathology such as myocardial infarct.**mitoxantrone** at a total dose of more than 140 mg/m2 can suffer congestive heart failure
- Anthracycline-induced cardiomyopathy.

Dysrhythmias:
- **dysrhythmias** unrelated to the cumulative dose
- Dysrhythmias may occur hours or even days after administration.
- Commonly observed dysrhythmias include supraventricular tachycardia, complete heart blocks, and ventricular tachycardia.
- Doxorubicin may prolong the QT interval.

- Anthracycline may enhance the myocardial depressive effect of anesthetics even in patients with normal resting cardiac function.

Cyclophosphamide causes myocardial tissue injury

A **cyclophosphamide** dose range of more than 120mg.kg−1 over 2 days can result in severe congestive heart failure and hemorrhagic myocarditis, pericarditis, and necrosis.

Busulfan oral daily dosage may suffer endocardia fibrosis, with signs and symptoms of constrictive cardiomyopathy.

Patients with preexisting cardiac disease receiving interferon in conventional doses may have exacerbations of their underlying illness.

 Mitomycin for extended periods of time and dosages has been shown to produce myocardial damage.

Paclitaxel, with cisplatinum, may also produce ventricular tachycardia

The preoperative and anesthetic assessment

- 2D-echocardiogram or nuclear medicine studies.
- Measurement of the left ventricular ejection fraction and detection of regional and global myocardial dysfunction. Where congestive failure is discovered, the physician will have to treat it preoperatively.

Types of cardiac toxicity

Acute and Sub-acute cardio toxicity:

- It can occur immediately after a single dose or a course of anthracycline therapy.
- Acute toxicity commonly (40%) takes the form of ECG changes such as nonspecific ST-T changes, decreased QRS voltage, and QT prolongation
- Decreased R wave amplitude has been thought by some to signal development of chronic cardiomyopathy later, though it is not proved.
- Sinus tachycardia is the most common rhythm disturbance but a variety of arrhythmias, including ventricular, supraventricular, and junctional tachycardia, have been reported.
- Atrioventricular and bundle-branch block have.
- These changes occur at all dose intervals and except for decreased QRS voltage, resolve 1 to 2 months after cessation of the therapy.
- Sudden death may also occur, due to ventricular fibrillation.
- Rare cases of sub-acute cardio toxicity resulting in acute failure of the left ventricle, pericarditis or a fatal pericarditis-myocarditis syndrome, particularly in children, have been reported.
- If these patients recover they should not receive further treatment with anthracycline.

- In elderly patients with preexisting heart disease, congestive heart failure can occur, which is generally transient and responds to normal medical management.

Chronic or late cardio toxicity:

- Chronic cardio toxicity after anthracycline classically takes the form of cardiomyopathy. CXR review may reveal cardiomegaly.
- ECG changes occur with these agents and include non-specific ST-and T-wave changes, premature atrial and ventricular contractions, sinus tachycardia and low-voltage QRS complexes.
- Anthracycline cardio toxicity is a cumulative dose related phenomenon.
- The incidence of congestive heart failure secondary to anthracycline induced cardio toxicity increases with dose.
- The rapid increase in incidence of CHF after a dose of 550 mg/m2 has made it a popular empiric-limiting dose for doxorubicin-induced cardio toxicity.

Late onset cardio toxicity:

- Occult ventricular dysfunction, heart failure and arrhythmias occurring in previously asymptomatic patients more than a year after anthracycline therapy.
- Doxorubicin can cause subclinical myocardial injury during pre-adolescent years and this in later years retards appropriate growth of the myocardium during growth spurt.

<u>Anesthetic management:-</u>

- Invasive monitoring techniques
- Invasive arterial blood pressure recordings and a pulmonary artery catheterization may be necessary if significant myocardial impairment is present.
- Anthracycline treated patients under anaesthesia can develop acute intraoperative left ventricular failure refractory to β-adrenergic receptor agonists.
- Amrinone and sulmazole are the new class of cardiotonics with inotropic drugs useful in such conditions.

B) **<u>Pulmonary effects and complications of cancer chemotherapy</u>**

- 75% to 90% of pulmonary complications are secondary to infection.
- The cancer patient can suffer infectious complications secondary to chemotherapy (e.g., Bleomycin), thoracic radiation, and multiple pulmonary resections.
- respiratory failure in cancer patients requiring assisted mechanical ventilation is associated with a 75% mortality rate
- Pulmonary infiltrates seen on a routine chest radiograph is extensive; there are many causes for such infiltrates.
- Busulfan, cyclophosphamide, paclitaxel, etc., can lead to pulmonary complications. Bleomycin, an anti-tumor agent, producing lung damage.

Bleomycin pulmonary toxicity produced by have been described:

- About 0-40% patients are reported to develop pulmonary toxicity
- 11-30% patients will have non-lethal pulmonary fibrosis and the mortality associated with Bleomycin toxicity will range from 2-10%.

The risk factors for Bleomycin pulmonary toxicity

- Old age
- Accumulative dose >400-450 U
- Poor pulmonary reserves
- Radiotherapy
- Uremia, higher inspired oxygen concentrations
- Concomitantly administered other anticancer drugs

Mechanisms of pulmonary toxicity:

- the threshold dose level for the development of pulmonary disease is in the range of 400 to 450mg,
- Fatal pulmonary fibrosis has been reported with doses as low as 50mg.
- The mechanism of pulmonary toxicity associated with the use of bleomycin, is probably due to direct cytotoxicity and in patients receiving bleomycin, type I pneumocytes are replaced by type II pneumocytes.

- Continued exposure to bleomycin prevents reversion of type II to type I pneumocytes and further leads to meta-plasia of the type II cells to cuboidal epithelium.
- Further exposure prevents effective repair and fibro blasts and macrophages migrate into the interstitium and the alveoli.
- Another mechanism for bleomycin toxicity involves the production of superoxide and other free radical moieties, Cleave nuclear DNA.
- The production of these highly oxidizing radicals might be increased by the inspiration of fortified concentrations of oxygen.

Pathology of chemotherapy pulmonary toxicity

- Dose dependent interstitial pneumonitis progressing to chronic fibrosis
- An acute hypersensitivity pneumonitis with peripheral eosinophilia resembling eosinophilic pneumonia.
- An acute chest pain syndrome.
- A bronchitis obliterans with organizing pneumonia.
- Pulmonary veno-occlusive disease.
- Progressive interstitial pneumonitis and fibrosis is the most common pattern of bleomycin lung injury.

Clinical picture of pulmonary toxicity

- Symptoms generally occur between 4 to 10 weeks after bleomycin therapy,
- 20% patients with radiographic and histological features of bleomycin toxicity may be present without any clinical symptoms.

.

Clinical presentation:

- The lesions seen frequently are in the lower lobes and sub pleural areas and chest X-ray shows bilateral basal and peri-hilar infiltrates with fibrosis.
- The first signs and symptoms of toxicity are fever, cough, dyspnea and bibasilar rhonchi and rales, which may progress to exertional dyspnea with mild X-ray changes and a normal restin PaO2or a severe form of hypoxia at rest.
- The earliest detection of pulmonary fibrosis may be achieved through the serial evaluation of pulmonary function.
- Sequential measurement of carbon monoxide diffusion capacity (DLCO) may indicate the presence of occult pulmonary changes.
- Arterial hypoxemia is commonly found and spirometry reveals decreased lung volumes compatible with restrictive lung disease.
- Regression or amelioration of the toxic pulmonary pathology may occur with immediate cessation of therapy. Steroid therapy has been found to be effective in some cases.

- Non cardiogenic pulmonary edema, chronic pneumonitis and fibrosis, and hypersensitivity pneumonitis.

<u>Anesthetic management of pulmonary toxicity</u>:
- Importance to the anesthesiologist is the debate about the amount of oxygen to be administered to a patient coming up for surgery after being given bleomycin.
- Perioperative oxygen restriction is not necessary
- Perioperative fluid balance including transfusions as a significant predictor of postoperative pulmonary morbidity.
- The duration of surgery and post-chemotherapy forced vital capacity are significant predictive factors of procedure related pulmonary morbidity.
- On the basis of available data it seems prudent to reduce the concentration of inspired oxygen to the lowest level to maintain SpO2 > 90%.
- Use of intraoperative PEEP to enhance oxygenation
- Fluid balance is another important factor in predicting pulmonary morbidity in-patients receiving bleomycin.
- Conservative fluid management is important; use of colloids is beneficial as compared to crystalloid.

<u>Intraoperative monitoring</u>

Arterial blood gas analysis should be performed by an indwelling arterial cannula or intermittent sampling.

Post-operative care

Postoperative use of rigorous physiotherapy to treat ventilation-perfusion abnormalities may

Effects of cancer chemotherapy agents on hepato-renal, and CNS system

Renal complications:-

- Cisplatinum, a commonly used anticancer drug has been found to produce toxic effects like nephrotoxicity, myelo suppression, neuropathy in stocking and glove distribution, auditory and visual impairment.
- The dose-limiting factor for single agent use, however, is nephrotoxicity. 30% of patients receiving cisplatinum will develop nephrotoxicity, especially if the hydration is not properly controlled.

Mechanism of renal complications of chemotherapy

- It causes coagulation necrosis of proximal and distal renal tubular epithelial cells and in the collecting ducts leading to are reduction in the renal blood flow and glomerular filtration rate (GFR).
- Cisplatinum leads to wasting of magnesium and potassium. A single dose of 2mg/kg or 50-75mg/m2 will produce nephrotoxicity in 25-30% of patients.

- The newer analogues of cisplatinum, such as carboplatinum and oxaloplatinum are less nephrotoxic with equal efficacy in controlling the malignancy.
- Methotrexate causes the acute nephrotoxicity as a result of its intratubular precipitation

Acute renal failure

- **Acute renal failure** can result within 24 hours of administration of a single dose of cisplatinum.
- Use of normal saline is particularly beneficial as high chloride concentrations in the tubules inhibit the hydrolysis of cisplatinum.
- The renal toxicity may be accentuated if the patient receives aminoglycosides concomitantly.

CNS complications:-

- Vinca alkaloids were the first anticancer drugs found to have neurotoxic effects. Vincristine is probably the only drug whose dose limiting toxicity is neurotoxicity.
- It can affect the central, peripheral or the autonomic nervous systems. Peripheral neuropathies present as peripheral paresthesia with depression of deep tendon reflexes.
- The paresthesia progress proximally with therapy. Motor dysfunction and gait disorders can occur.
- Vincristine, vinblastine, procarbazine, cisplatinum
- All can cause a toxic neuropathy with paresthesia, loss of deep tendon reflexes and muscle weakness.

- Autonomic neuropathy with orthostatic hypotension is a rare concomitant of neoplasia
- Cranial nerve effects may manifest as opthalmoplegia and facial palsy
- Autonomic neuropathy can present as orthostatic hypotension, erectile dysfunction, constipation, difficulty in micturition, bladder atony, et
- **Cisplatinum**, along with its effects on the kidney also affects the nervous system. 50% patients receiving cisplatinum will display neurotoxicity depending on dose and treatment duration. It generally takes the form of paresthesias.
- Continued treatment will lead to loss of deep tendon reflexes, vibration sense and sensory ataxia.

Regional anesthesia and neuropathy

- Regional anesthesia is concerned, one should be aware that in a considerable percentage of patients a sub-clinical, unrecognized neuropathy may be present in patients with previous cisplatinum chemotherapy.
- Recently, a diffuse brachial plexopathy after interscalene blockade has been reported in a patient receiving cisplatinum chemotherapy.
- Thus, if regional anaesthesia is contemplated, a detailed pre-operative neurological examination.

Hepatic complications:-

- Hepatocellular dysfunction is manifested as raised serum enzymes,
- Fatty infiltration of liver and cholestasis, due to direct toxic effect of the drug or its metabolite.
- L-asparginase and cytarabine are most commonly implicated agents in hepatocellular dysfunction.
- A decreased synthetic function with low proteins and coagulation abnormalities may be seen. Ascites, painful hepatomegaly, and encephalopathy may result after administration of cytarabine, cyclophosphamide, mitomycin, etc.

Hematological complications:-

- Bone marrow function in cancer patients may be disturbed by primary bone marrow disorders (e.g., leukemia), bony metastases (e.g., from breast cancer), as well as myelosuppressive chemotherapy.
- The production of any or all blood elements may be impaired. There is dysfunctional coagulation. The PT and PTT are shortened. There is increase in factor I, V, VIII, IX, XI and FDP.
- There is reduced survival of the platelets and the decreased antithrombin III activity.
- Some investigators have maintained a minimal level of 50,000 platelets per microliter in the intraoperative and postoperative period. Correction of other coagulation

disturbances is important before undertaking surgical intervention in the thrombocytopenic patient.

- Close cooperation among the surgeon, anesthesiologist, and hematologistis required for optimal management and maximal safety.
- Myelo-suppression caused by all the chemotherapeutic agents is partially or completely reversible within 1 to 6 weeks of termination of therapy.

Syndrome of inappropriate antidiuretic hormone secretion (SIADH):-

- Another metabolic abnormality in patients with cancer like lung, pancreas-adeno-carcinoma, duodenum, thymoma, mesothelioma, leukaemia, Hodgkin, reticulum cell sarcoma, is SIADH, which occurs in 1% to2% of cancer patients.
- Some drugs, such as vasopressin, carbamazepine, oxytocin, vincristine, vinblastine, cyclophosphamide, phenothizianes, tricyclic antidepressant agents, narcotics, and monoamine oxidase inhibitors, can also induce SIADH.

Steroid administration:

- The oncology patient often has a history of exogenous glucocorticoid administration as part of a chemotherapy regimen.
- The physician at the time of pre-operative evaluation has to decide on the use and the amount of stress steroid coverage.

- The patient who has received ≥2 weeks of glucocorticoids within the past year is considered at risk for adrenal suppression.
- However, many of these patients are capable of a normal stress response. The corticotrophin (ACTH) stimulation test is the definitive test to identify adrenal suppression.

Tumorlysis syndrome:-

- Chemotherapy induces rapid tumor cell lysis in patients with a large malignant cell burden over an exquisitely sensitive tumor
- This classically occurs in patients with Burkitt's lymphoma, non-Hodgkin's lymphomas, acute lymphoblastic and non-lymphoblastic leukemias, and chronic myelogenous leukemia

- In addition, it may also occur continuously in patients with lymphomas and leukemia following treatment with chemotherapy, radiation, glucocorticoids, tamoxifen, or interferon. The clinical manifestations of this syndrome are related to the metabolic abnormalities.
- In those patients with suspected tumor lysis syndrome or for those patients who receive chemotherapeutic agents likely to induce the syndrome, prevention is the mainstay of treatment.
- To prevent the development of acute renal failure, patients who are to undergo treatment for malignancies should receive vigorous intravenous hydration, often with diuretics or renal doses of dopamine to ensure adequate urine output

Chemotherapy and wound healing:-

- The outcome of surgical procedures may be affected by the wound-healing impairment caused by antineoplastic agents used to treat the underlying tumor. The neutropenia that accompanies some chemotherapy within 7 to 10 days of administration can interfere with the early phases of wound healing.

- The effects of chemotherapy directly on wound healing depend on dose and the timing of drug administration relative to creation of the wound.

- A high incidence of wound complications has been reported in women undergoing mastectomy after receiving preoperative chemotherapy and radiation. Bleomycin has not been associated with increased wound complications.

Preoperative risk assessment

1) type of surgery

Breast cancer surgery low risk

Intrabdominal (colorectal), and intrathoracic lung cancer are intermediate risk

2.Ischemic heart disease
Preoperative evaluation of ischemic heart disease

- Perioperative myocardial infarction (MI) is a major cause of morbidity and mortality in patients who have noncardiac surgery

- **Stress testing should be reserved for patients at moderate to high risk undergoing moderate- or high-risk surgery and those who have poor exercise capacity.**

- **Further cardiovascular studies should be limited to patients who are at high risk, have poor exercise tolerance, or have known poor ventricular function.**

- **Medical therapy using beta blockers, statins, and alpha agonists may be effective in high-risk patients.**

- **statins and alpha agonists, whether or not these therapies are as effective in patients with subclinical coronary artery disease or left ventricular dysfunction, and the optimal timing and dosing regimens of these medications.**

- American College of Cardiology/American Heart Association (ACC/AHA) Guidelines on Perioperative Cardiovascular Evaluation for Noncardiac Surgery provide an evidence-based approach to perioperative evaluation and management of these patients; these guidelines were updated in 2002.[2]

Cardiac risk factor for perioperative myocardial infarction

Major

- Unstable coronary syndromes
- Acute or recent* MI with evidence of important ischemic risk by clinical symptoms or noninvasive study
- Unstable or severe† angina (Canadian class III or IV‡)
- Decompensated heart failure
- High-grade atrioventricular block
- Symptomatic ventricular arrhythmias in the presence of underlying heart disease
- Supraventricular arrhythmias with uncontrolled ventricular rate
- Severe valvular disease
- Mild angina pectoris (Canadian class I or II‡)

Intermediate

- Previous MI by history or pathologic Q waves
- Compensated or prior heart failure
- Diabetes mellitus (particularly insulin-dependent)
- Renal insufficiency

Minor

- Advanced age (older than 75 years)
- Abnormal electrocardiography results (e.g., left ventricular hypertrophy, left bundle branch block, ST-T abnormalities
- Rhythm other than sinus (e.g., atrial fibrillation)
- Low functional capacity (e.g., inability to climb one flight of stairs with a bag of groceries)

- History of stroke

- Uncontrolled systemic hypertension

Preoperative Cardiac Assessment

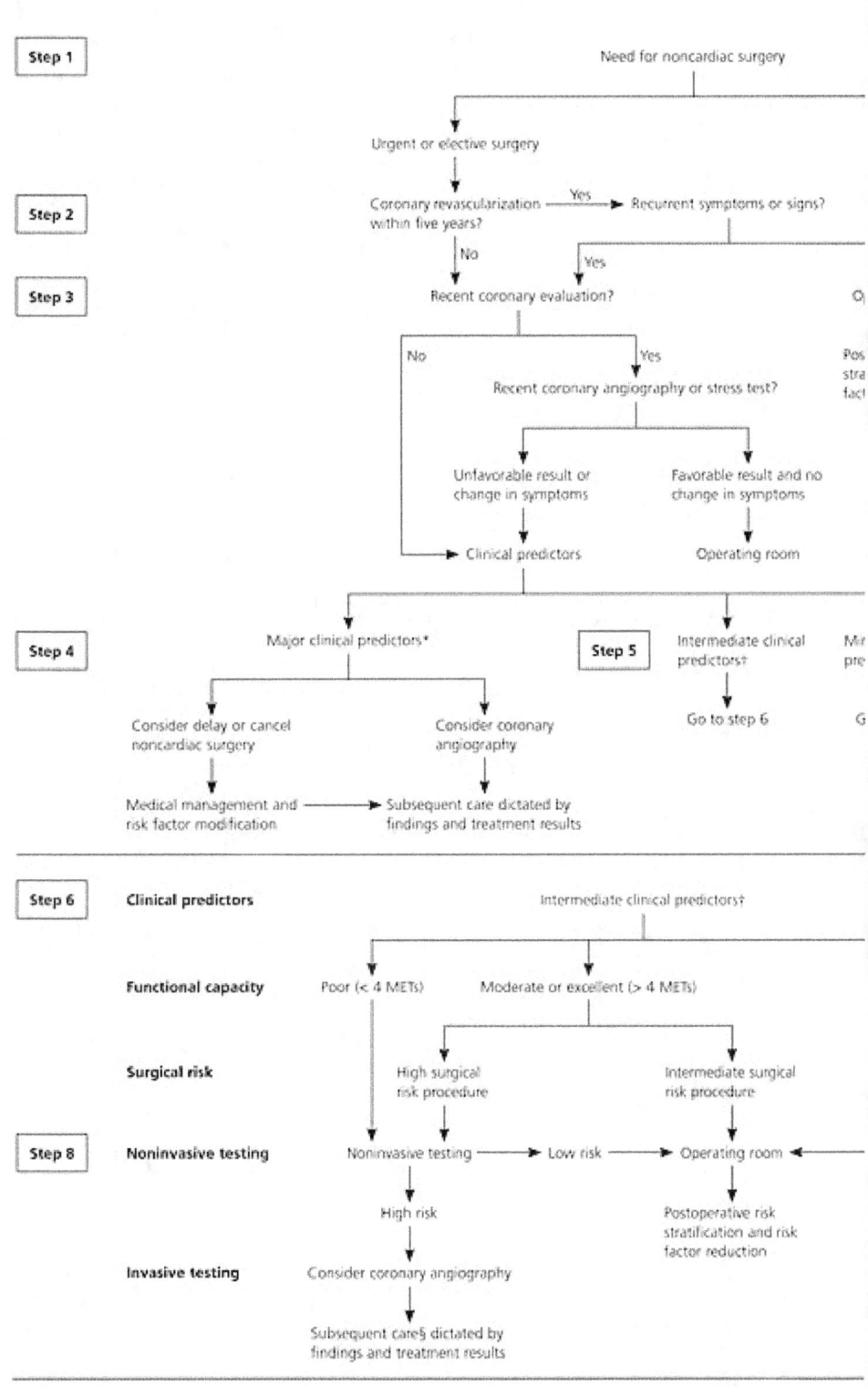

Step 1

Need for noncardiac surgery

Urgent or elective surgery

Step 2

Coronary revascularization ——Yes——▶ Recurrent symptoms or signs?
within five years?

No   Yes

Step 3

Recent coronary evaluation?   O

No   Yes   Pos
                                                                 stra
                     Recent coronary angiography or stress test? fact

Unfavorable result or   Favorable result and no
change in symptoms   change in symptoms

              Clinical predictors   Operating room

Step 4

Major clinical predictors*   **Step 5** Intermediate clinical   Mir
                                                predictors†   pre

Consider delay or cancel   Consider coronary   Go to step 6   G
noncardiac surgery   angiography

Medical management and ——▶ Subsequent care dictated by
risk factor modification   findings and treatment results

Step 6 **Clinical predictors**   Intermediate clinical predictors†

Functional capacity   Poor (< 4 METs)   Moderate or excellent (> 4 METs)

Surgical risk   High surgical   Intermediate surgical
                                 risk procedure   risk procedure

Step 8 **Noninvasive testing**   Noninvasive testing ——▶ Low risk ——▶ Operating room ◀——

                                 High risk   Postoperative risk
                                                              stratification and risk
Invasive testing   Consider coronary angiography   factor reduction

                   Subsequent care§ dictated by
                   findings and treatment results

Step 7 **Clinical predictors**   Minor or no clinical predictors‡

Lee's Revised Cardiac Risk Index

CLINICAL VARIABLE

High-risk surgery (i.e., intraperitoneal, intrathoracic, or suprainguinal vascular surgery)

Coronary artery disease

Congestive heart failure

History of cerebrovascular disease

Insulin treatment for diabetes mellitus

Preoperative serum creatinine level greater than 2.0 mg per dL (180 μmol per L)

BETA BLOCKERS

- Beta blockers should be given peri operatively to patients with known ischemic heart disease undergoing vascular surgery or who have previously taken beta blockers.

- Beta blockers generally are not recommended for patients with low to moderate risk of perioperative cardiovascular complications.

- Statin use is associated with a reduction in perioperative risk in patients with pre-existing coronary artery disease, although randomized trial data are lacking.

- Alpha$_2$-agonists such as clonidine (Catapres) are a possible alternative to beta blockers to reduce perioperative risk of cardiac complications in high-risk patients.

Preoperative preparation of congestive heart failure:

- .Surgery should be delayed in patients with decompensated or untreated cardiomyopathy.

- Preoperative evaluation requires combined approach of anesthesiologists, cardiologist and surgeons

- Patients with dilated and hypertrophic cardiomyopathy are prone to the development of congestive heart failure in the perioperative period.

- Preoperative evaluation includes history, physical examination, ECG, chest radiography, complete blood count, electrolytes, creatinine, glomerular filtration rate, glucose, liver enzymes, urine analysis, BNP and echocardiographic evaluation of left ventricular function. Drug therapy should be optimized and continued preoperatively.

2. Preoperative preparation of cerebrovascular disease

- Patients with a history of stroke or TIA are at increased risk for perioperative stroke after major cardiac and vascular surgical procedures

- Patients with few risk factors for perioperative stroke undergoing low-risk noncardiac surgery do not need further testing.

Stroke history and planned cardiac procedure, including aortic manipulation, performing a transesophageal echocardiography to identify aortic atherosclerotic plaques should be considered.

Perioperative strokes are predominantly embolic, and are related in large part to perioperative atrial fibrillation, especially after cardiac procedures.

Preoperative initiation of amiodarone or ß-blockers may decrease the incidence of postoperative atrial fibrillation and stroke.

Antithrombotic

- They are widely used for secondary stroke prevention. Abrupt discontinuation of antiplatelet agents before surgery may be associated with increased risk for stroke recurrence due to rebound hypercoagulability.

- Aspirin should be stopped only 2 to 3 days before major neurosurgical procedures. Continuation of aspirin therapy is acceptable during regional spinal anesthesia, nerve blocks, dermatological cutaneous surgeries, dental procedures, ophthalmological procedures, peripheral vascular procedures, cardiac surgeries, and endoscopies.[

- Clopidogrel, on the other hand, appears unsafe and should be discontinued 5 to 7 days before surgical procedures.

-] There are no studies regarding the safety of dipyridamole, alone or in combination with aspirin, during surgery. It is therefore prudent to withhold it 5 to 7 days preoperatively.

- Substituting clopidogrel and dipyridamole with aspirin in patients at high risk for stroke during the preoperative period.

- For many patients taking warfarin for stroke prevention, the risk of perioperative discontinuation of anticoagulation exceeds the risk of bleeding complications. Preoperative bridging therapy with heparin is advised and warfarin is discontinued. Heparin can be stopped hours prior to the procedure and warfarin restarted 24 hours after surgery.

- Preoperative assessment of stroke patients should ensure that blood pressure is adequately controlled throughout the perioperative period.

Preoperative preparation of insulin dependent patient.

- using general management principles to minimize the likelihood of hypoglycemia and to limit the incidence of excessive hyperglycemia
- For these patients, short-acting insulin may be administered subcutaneously on a sliding scale or as a continuous infusion,

to maintain optimal glucose control, depending on the type and duration of surgery.

- Patients who are insulin dependent are typically advised to reduce their bedtime dose of insulin the night before surgery to prevent hypoglycemia while nil per os (NPO).

- Maintenance insulin may be continued, based on the history of glucose concentrations and the discretion of the advising clinician.

- Patients may be advised to consult with their anesthesiologist and diabetes-managing practitioner for individualized recommendations regarding their diabetes plan.

- Additionally, patients should be monitored preoperatively to assess for hyperglycemia and hypoglycemia.

- Intravenous insulin is the most flexible and readily titratable agent, making it an ideal modality for perioperative use.

- The length of surgery, the type of surgery, and the degree of glycemic dysregulation dictate the amount of supplemental insulin.

- For patients with type 1 DM, it is recommended to schedule elective surgeries as the first case of the day to minimally disrupt their DM regimen. Depending on the length and the extent of surgery, patients may be advised to administer one half of their daily dose of long-acting insulin and to arrive at the preoperative admitting area early enough to have their serum glucose monitored and to determine whether they need intravenous dextrose until the time of surgery.

- Establish separate intravenous access for a "piggyback" infusion of **regular insulin** (100 U per 100 mL 0.9% saline). The infusion rate can be determined by using the following formula: insulin (U/hr) = serum glucose (mg/dL)/150. Intra-arterial catheter placement is recommended to facilitate checking blood glucose concentrations every 1-2 hours intraoperatively and postoperatively.
- A second intravenous catheter may be used for intravascular volume replacement with a normal saline solution

Postoperative management of diabetic patient

- Postoperatively, diabetic patients present unique challenges. Initiation of nutrition is often delayed and frequently interrupted for diagnostic studies or procedures.
- To reduce the likelihood of adverse effects, the regimen selected should accommodate ongoing changes and reflect the patient's current clinical status.
- These include nutritional feeding (continuous vs intermittent), severity of illness, and corticosteroid and catecholamine use

4. Preoperative preparation of patient with creatinine more than 2

- The administration of **general anesthesia** may induce a reduction in renal blood flow in up to 50% of patients, resulting in the impaired excretion of nephrotoxic drugs.

- In addition, the function of cholinesterase, an enzyme responsible for breaking down certain anesthetic agents, may be impaired, resulting in

- Prolonged respiratory muscle paralysis if neuromuscular blocking agents are used.

- N -acetyl-procainamide, a metabolite of procainamide, accumulates in persons with chronic kidney disease (CKD) and, when used in combination with histamine-2 (H2) blockers, causes prolongation of the QT. The dose of procainamide should be adjusted, or a substitute should be used.

- Fluorinated compounds, such as methoxyflurane and enflurane, are nephrotoxic and should be avoided in patients with CKD. Succinylcholine, a depolarizing blocker, causes hyperkalaemia.

Complication Prevention

Hyperkalemia

- tissue breakdown,

- transfusions

- acidosis,

- ACE inhibitors

- beta-blockers

- heparin,

- rhabdomyolysis,

- Ringer lactate solution as a replacement fluid.

- Ringer lactate solution contains potassium, which is often disregarded but can cause hyperkalemia.

- Third-space fluid loss, diarrhoea, vomiting, and nasoenteric suction result in both volume contraction and hypokalemia.

Hypokalaemia is sometimes followed concomitantly with hypomagnesaemia.

acidosis

Most patients with CKD have chronic acidosis; surgical disease can further complicate the acidemia. Such patients are at a higher risk for hyperkalaemia, myocardial depression, and cardiac arrhythmia.

Hypocalcemia and hyperphosphatemia may be caused by rhabdomyolysis. Hyponatraemia may occur from hypotonic fluids or inappropriate secretion of antidiuretic hormone.

Brain tumor with pregnancy

Introduction

Brain tumor surgery during pregnancy has a great concern in Egypt now days. High prevalence of brain tumors during pregnancy y was noticed. There is no accurate statics for the prevalence. The most common tumors are pituitary tumors, meningioma, gliomas, and metastis of breast carcinomas. Many problems affects anesthesia, as the interaction between many different factors, as the physiological changes during pregnancy, including, cardiovascular, respiratory Changes. Problems occur, during diagnosis, and treatment of tumors. Also problems during surgery are, drug interactions with the anesthesia drugs, blood loss and transfusion, prevention preterm labor, and anesthesia for urgent cesarean section during surgery for removal of brain tumor, in the chapter I tried to summary all these factors from anesthesia point of views did many cases for brain resection during pregnancy, I hope to give this experience for any young anesthesia how may facing such cases

Common tumors during pregnancy

Meningiomas

The incidence of meningiomas is approximately twice as high in women as in men. Specifically, intracranial meningiomas are twice as common and intra spinal meningiomas nine times as common in females. Meningiomas also seem to have a relationship to sex hormones with accelerated growth of these tumors during the luteal phase of the menstrual cycle and during pregnancy. There may also be an increased incidence of meningiomas in women with breast cancer, although one study contests this relationship. A large number of studies have examined the role of androgen, estrogen and progesterone receptors in meningiomas with most finding progesterone and androgen receptors in a high proportion and low levels of estrogen receptors in a small proportion of meningioma specimens obtained at the time of initial surgery and at recurrence

Pituitary tumors

Pituitary tumors account for approximately 15% of all primary intracranial neoplasms and occur in higher frequency in women, mainly in the child-bearing years. The female preponderance of these tumors is due to the increased frequency of prolactinomas in women in the second and third decades. Women are affected four times as commonly as men and account for 78% of all prolactinomas.

1.2. Cranial metastases

Breast cancer

Breast cancer is the most common malignancy among women in North America accounting for 27% of all cancers. Approximately 181,000 new cases of breast cancer were diagnosed in

1992 and 46,000 women died from the disease the same year. Neurologic complications occur in approximately 25% of patients with metastatic breast cancer although autopsy studies have demonstrated central nervous system involvement in 31-57% of examinations.

2. Problems in management of brain tumors with pregnancy
2.1. Problems in diagnosis

Symptoms of increased intracranial pressure including headache, nausea and vomiting are similar to the symptoms of early pregnancy, or pregnancy related hypertensive diseases (eclampsia or preeclampsia).

The use of Neuro imaging of the pregnant patient with these symptoms become necessary. In the first trimester it is preferred to be avoided. The MRI is the procedure of choice as there is no exposure to ionizing radiation. Although there is no evidence that MRI affects the fetus there is exposure to powerful electromagnetic fields and this imaging modality should be avoided if possible in the first trimester. Similarly, there is very little evidence regarding the safety of the ferromagnetic contrast agent gadolinium and this is not sanctioned for use in pregnancy and should be avoided if possible. In the patient with rapid neurologic deterioration computerized tomography (CT) may be necessary. This does involve radiation exposure of approximately

2.5 to 3 rads to the head of the patient and a fetal exposure estimated to be approximately 1 m rad or less per slice which can be reduced by appropriate shielding of the uterus with a lead apron. At fetal exposures less than 10 rads no adverse effects in excess of the background rate of spontaneous abnormalities in 3% of live births and the spontaneous abortion rate of 30% in all pregnancies. Medically indicated exposures of up to 5 rads are considered acceptable in pregnancy when unavoidable. There has been limited experience

556 Clinical Management and Evolving Novel Therapeutic Strategies for Patients with Brain Tumors with the use of iodinated contrast agents during pregnancy and the risks are not precisely defined. Such agents should be avoided in the first trimester.

Problems during treatment

Treatment of brain tumors or their complications may be necessary during pregnancy. Cerebral edema and increased intracranial pressure may require the use of glucocorticoids and mannitol. Glucocorticoids have been used during pregnancy for other reasons including the prevention of neonatal respiratory distress syndrome and there is no evidence of growth, physical, motor or developmental deficiencies within the first three years of life. However, fetal adrenal suppression may occur with long-term, high dose therapy during any part of pregnancy and necessitates the use of supplemental steroids in the peri-partum period. Although mannitol does cross the placenta and is excreted by the fetal kidney into the amniotic fluid no adverse effects have been reported.

Cranial irradiation exposes the fetus to higher doses of radiation than diagnostic imaging. In general, radiation exposure in utero carries a risk of adverse fetal outcomes including spontaneous abortion, anatomic malformation, growth and mental retardation and possibly childhood cancer with the latter risk highest in the first trimester The exposure to the fetus from scatter is low when conventional radiation therapy is delivered to parts distant from the uterus and such exposure carries low risk. Strategies to reduce fetal exposure include the use of focal rather than whole brain irradiation, radiation dose reduction, substitution of heavy charged particles for photons and deferring radiation until after delivery.

Chemotherapy typically involves agents which are teratogenic in the first trimester and associated with adverse fetal outcomes. Properties of chemotherapeutic agents which improve permeability across the blood brain barrier also facilitate transport across the placenta making these drugs especially hazardous. Although there is data to suggest that certain chemotherapeutic agents are associated with minimal risk in the second and third trimesters, chemotherapy for malignant brain tumors should be avoided during pregnancy. Meningiomas are tumors that are thought to arise from meningothelial cells which make up the arachnoid villi of the meninges. These lesions account for approximately 20% of all intracranial and 25% of all intra spinal tumors and the incidence increases with age

Problems during anesthesia for brain tumor surgery

Altered maternal physiology.

Respiratory system and acid-base balance changes

a. Alveolar ventilation increases 25% by the fourth month of gestation and 45% to 70% by term. This results in a chronic respiratory alkalosis, with a Paco2 of 28 to 32 mm Hg, a slightly alkaline pH (e.g., approximately 7.44), and decreased levels of bicarbonate and buffer base.

b. oxygen consumption increases during gestation, Pao2 usually increases slightly or remains within the normal range.

c. Functional residual capacity (FRC) decreases by approximately 20% as the uterus expands, which results in decreased oxygen reserve and the potential for airway closure.

d. obesity; perioperative intra-abdominal distention; placement of the patient in the supine,

Trendelenburg, or lithotomy positions), airway closure may be sufficient to cause hypoxemia

e. Failed intubation (which is the leading cause of maternal death from anesthesia) is as much

a risk during non-obstetric surgery as it is during cesarean section.

f. rapid development of hypoxemia and acidosis during periods of hypoventilation or apnea due to decreased FRC, increased oxygen consumption, and diminished buffering capacity.

g. induction of general anesthesia occurs more rapidly during pregnancy, because alveolar hyperventilation and a decreased FRC allow faster equilibration of inhaled agents.

h. Acceleration in the induction of anesthesia is the approximately 30% decrease in the minimum alveolar concentration (MAC) for volatile anesthetic agents that occurs even during early gestation.

Cardiovascular system changes

a. Cardiac output increases by 30% to 50% during pregnancy because of increases in heart rate and stroke volume; both systemic and pulmonary vascular resistance decrease.

b. By eight weeks' gestation, 57% of the increase in cardiac output, 78% of the increase in stroke volume, and 90% of the decrease in systemic vascular resistance that typically are achieved by 24 weeks' gestation.

c. During the second half of gestation, the weight of the uterus compresses the inferior vena cava when the mother lies supine; this decreases venous return and cardiac output by approximately 25% to 30%.

d. Although upper extremity blood pressure may be maintained by compensatory vasoconstriction and tachycardia, uteroplacental perfusion is jeopardized whenever the mother lies supine.

e. Frank hypotension also can occur in the supine parturient, especially when regional or general anesthesia attenuates or abolishes normal compensatory mechanisms. It is essential to displace the uterus laterally during any operation performed after the twentieth week of pregnancy.

Factors that can alter uteroplacental blood flow

1. Uterine Contraction

2. Decreased Uterine Blood Flow

3. Pathological Conditions

4. Pharmacological Agents

558 Clinical Management and Evolving Novel Therapeutic
Strategies for Patients with Brain Tumors

Intravenous induction agents

5. Inhalation agents (Desflurane and Sevoflurane)

6. Antihypertensive agents

7. b-adrenergic blocking drugs

8. Tocolytic drugs

9. Epidural and subarachnoid opiates

10. Local anesthetics

11. Pharmacological agent added to the local anesthetic

12. Vasopressors

Maintenance of uteroplacental blood flow is the hallmark for fetal well-being; hence an in depth knowledge of this subjects essential for individuals taking care of pregnant women.

Uterine blood flow is determined by the equation. Hence any condition that will significantly decrease mean uterine arterial pressure – Uterine venous pressure

Uterine vascular resistance

So when maternal arterial pressure decreases or significantly increase uterine vascular resistance will decrease utero placental blood flow and, ultimately, umbilical blood flow. At term, 10% of the cardiac output (700 mL/min) supplies the uterus. The placental vasculature remains maximally.

Changes in blood volume and blood constituents

• Blood volume expands in the first trimester and increases 30% to 45% by term. A smaller increase in red blood cell volume than in plasma volume results in a dilutional anemia.

• Moderate blood loss is well tolerated during pregnancy, preexisting anemia decreases the patient's reserve when significant hemorrhage occurs. Fresh blood transfusion is needed to compensate blood loss during brain tumor surgery.

• Pregnancy induces a hypercoagulable state, with increases in fibrinogen; factors VII, VIII,

X, and XII; and fibrin degradation products. Pregnancy is associated with enhanced platelet turnover, clotting, and fibrinolysis, and there is a wide range in the normal platelet count; thus pregnancy represents a state of accelerated but compensated intravascular coagulation.

During the postoperative period, pregnant surgical patients are at high risk for thromboembolic

Complications.

• It is great challenge to induce hypotensive technique and to maintain the placental perfusion pressure.

Gastrointestinal system changes

• Incompetence of the lower esophageal sphincter and distortion of gastric and pyloric anatomy result in an increased risk of esophageal reflux and aspiration pneumonitis.

• It seems prudent to consider any pregnant patient at risk for aspiration after 18 to 20 weeks' gestation.

• Rapid sequence induction to avoid aspiration and deep anesthesia to prevent increase in the intracranial pressure during brain tumor surgery is another problem.

• Preoperative antiacid, sodium citreate, metoclopramide, muscle relaxant as Rocuronium.

• Complete recovery is needed before extubation.

Altered Responses to Anesthesia

• The decrease in MAC for inhaled anesthetic agents,

• Thiopental requirements begin to decrease early in pregnancy.

• Plasma cholinesterase levels decrease by approximately 25% from early in pregnancy until the seventh postpartum day. Cautions in use of remifentanil and succinylcholine.

• *The anesthesiologist should monitor neuromuscular blockade with a nerve sti*mulator to ensure adequate reversal before extubation.

• Decreased protein binding associated with low albumin concentrations during pregnancy may result in a greater fraction of unbound drug, with the potential for greater drug toxicity during pregnancy.

• Antiepileptic drugs as **Carbamazepine** and, Phenytoin may potentiate effects of anesthetic drug used.

Risk of teratogenicity

• *Teratogenicity* has been defined as any significant postnatal change in function or form in an offspring after prenatal treatment. Concern about the potential harmful effects of anesthetic agents stems from their known effects on mammalian cells. These occur at clinical concentrations and include reversible decreases in cell motility, prolongation of DNA synthesis, and inhibition of cell division .Despite these theoretical concerns, no data specifically link any of these cellular events with teratogenic changes.

Anticonvulsants

• All anticonvulsants cross the placenta. Pregnant women with epilepsy who ingest anticonvulsant drugs have a fetal congenital anomaly rate of 4% to 8%, which is higher than the 2% to 3% background incidence quoted for the general population.

• **Carbamazepine**

• **Phenobarbital** is used in the treatment of partial and generalized tonic-clonic seizures and status epilepticus

• **Valproic acid** (Depakene, Depakote) is used to treat absence and generalized tonic-clonic seizures.

• Tranquilizers

Some studies have suggested that first-trimester exposure to diazepam increases the risk of cleft lip.

Lithium

In the International Registry of Lithium Babies, (11.5%) of 217 infants exposed to lithium during the first trimester of pregnancy were malformed. Eighteen infants had cardiovascular anomalies.

Antidepressants

The selective serotonin reuptake inhibitors include sertraline (Zoloft), paroxetine (Paxil), fluoxetine (Prozac), and citalopram (Celexa). No increased risk of major malformations or developmental (language and behavior) abnormalities has been identified.

Nitrous oxide

In vivo and embryo culture studies in rats have confirmed that nitrous oxide produces several adverse reproductive effects, each of which results from exposure at a specific period of susceptibility. Use of electronic fetal monitoring for assessing fetal well-being has become universal, used by both physicians and nurses. Monitoring the fetal heart rate is used to determine adequate cerebral oxygenation of the fetus. As the brain modulates the heart, a decrease in fetal heart rate is believed to reflect inadequate fetal cerebral oxygenation. External fetal heart rate monitors use a Doppler detective device with computerized logic to interpret, and count the Doppler signals, whereas internal fetal heart rate monitors involve placement of an electrode on the fetal scalp. The presence of fetal heart tones as well as their rate and rhythm are well-recognized indicators of fetal well-being. A normal fetal .heart rate tracing reveals a rate of 110–160 beats/min with minimal to moderate beat-to beat variability with or without accelerations. A preterm fetus is expected to have a more rapid rate with little or no beat-to-beat variability and no accelerations (an increase in fetal heart rate over baseline, usually occurring with fetal movement.

The goal of antepartum fetal surveillance is to document fetal wellbeing, allowing the pregnancy to continue without concern for fetal death. Several antepartum techniques in use include fetal movement, nonstress test, contraction stress test, biophysical profile, and umbilical artery Doppler flow velocimetry.

Prevention of preterm labor

Fetal movement is the easiest means for documenting fetal wellbeing. The mother can perceive fetal movements, which serve as a basis for assessment. A diminution in the perception of fetal movement often precedes fetal death. Perception of 10 distinct movements in a period of up to 2 hours is considered reassuring. Heart rate reactivity is thought to be a good indicator of normal fetal autonomic function. Loss of reactivity is associated most commonly with fetal sleep but also may result from any central nervous system depression. A nonstress test involves connecting them other to the fetal heart rate monitor and observing. Non stress test results can be categorized as reactive or nonreactive.

The non-stress test is considered *reactive* (normal) if two or more fetal heart rate accelerations are observed within a 20-minute period. The non-stress test is considered *nonreactive* when no accelerations are observed.

Guidelines for the management of preterm delivery.

• Confirm diagnosis of preterm labor

• Exclude contraindications to expectant management and/or tocolysis

• Administer corticosteroids, if indicated

• Group B *Streptococcus* chemoprophylaxis, if indicated

• Pharmacologic tocolysis

• Consider transfer to tertiary care center

There is increased incidence of abortion and preterm delivery. Volatile halogenated agents depress myometrial irritability, the prophylactic use of tocolytic agents is controversial; they are not without risk, and it is unclear whether they affect outcome. Selective administration to those patients at greatest risk (e.g., those undergoing cervical cerclage) has been suggested

Anesthetic management

1. Unlike other operations wherein the patient is primarily concerned with him or herself, the pregnant woman usually is concerned for her baby's welfare.

2. The anesthesia provider must be aware of the various physiologic changes of pregnancy and incorporate them into the anesthetic plan.

3. These physiologic changes have implications for various diseases and must be considered.

4. The central nervous system effect of pregnancy include a reduced local anesthetic requirement when these agents are given intrathecally or epidurally.

5. Pregnant patients are at increased risk for aspiration during general anesthesia.

6. There is some suggestion that surgery during the first trimester is linked to central nervous

Defects during surgery.

7. Fetal heart rate monitoring is possible during some surgical procedures but is not universally used in the United States.

8. Preterm delivery remains the leading cause of perinatal morbidity and mortality in the

United States. Preterm labor is difficult to control with medication; the most promising medications are the calcium channel-blocking drugs. Magnesium sulfate is frequently used and is associated with prolonged depolarizing and non-depolarizing neuromuscular blockade.

9. The etiology of preeclampsia remains to be elucidated but is believed to be triggered by a paternal antigen in a susceptible mother.

10. Magnesium sulfate is the most effective medication for the prevention of seizures in women with preeclampsia.

11. Labetalol is the preferred medication for the control of blood pressure in mothers with preeclampsia.

12. The two causes of antepartum hemorrhage are placenta previa and placental abruption.

Associated with the increase in cesarean sections is a high risk of placenta accreta in patients with placenta previa.

13. Perinatal transmission of HIV is low if the viral load is <1,000 copies/mL, and patients with these levels do not require cesarean section. If the viral load is greater, cesarean section may decrease the risk of perinatal transmission.

3. Preoperative management

Premedication may be necessary to allay maternal anxiety.

Precautions against acid aspiration should include administration of an H2-receptor antagonist and 30 mL of a clear antacid before the induction of anesthesia.

4. Choice of anesthesia

The choice of anesthesia should be guided by maternal indications and should take into consideration the site and the nature of the surgery. No study has correlated improved fetal outcome with any anesthetic technique. When possible, local or regional anesthesia (with the exception of par cervical block) is preferred; this permits the administration of drugs with no laboratory or clinical evidence of teratogenesis. In addition, maternal respiratory complications occur less frequently with local and regional anesthetic techniques. These techniques are suitable for cases involving cervical cerclage, urologic or lower extremity procedures, and operations on the arm or hand. Most abdominal operations require general anesthesia, because the incision typically extends to the upper abdomen, which creates an unacceptable risk of aspiration in a pregnant patient with an unprotected airway.

5. Prevention of aorto caval compression

Beginning at 18 to 20 weeks' gestation, the pregnant patient should be transported on her side, and the uterus should be displaced leftward when she is positioned on the operating table.

6. Monitoring

Maternal monitoring should include noninvasive or direct blood pressure measurement, electrocardiography, pulse oximetry, capnography, temperature monitoring, and the use of a nerve stimulator. The FHR and uterine activity should be monitored both during and after surgery when technically feasible.

7. Anesthetic technique

General anesthesia mandates endotracheal intubation beginning at approximately 18 to 20 weeks' gestation or earlier if gastrointestinal function is abnormal. De nitrogenation (i.e., pre oxygenation) should precede the application of cricoid pressure, rapid-sequence induction, and endotracheal intubation. Drugs with a history of safe use during pregnancy include thiopental, morphine, meperidine, fentanyl, succinylcholine, and most of the nondepolarizing muscle relaxants. Many obstetric anesthesiologists would now add propofol to the list of "safe" drugs for use during pregnancy.

A commonly used technique employs a high concentration of oxygen, a muscle relaxant, and an opioid and/or a moderate concentration of a volatile halogenated agent. Scientific evidence does not support avoiding nitrous oxide during pregnancy, particularly after the sixth week of gestation. Omission of nitrous oxide may increase fetal risk if inadequate anesthesia results or if a high dose of a volatile agent results in maternal hypotension. A cautious approach would restrict nitrous oxide administration to a concentration of 50% or less and would limit its use in extremely long operations. Hyperventilation should be avoided; rather, end-tidal CO_2 should be maintained in the normal range for pregnancy. Before the administration of spinal or epidural anesthesia, rapid intravenous infusion of 1 L of crystalloid seems prudent, although the anesthesiologist should not assume that this will prevent maternal hypotension. Appropriate vasopressors should be available to treat hypotension if it occurs. The usual precautions must be taken to guard against a high block and systemic local anesthetic toxicity.

Regardless of the technique used, avoidance of hypoxemia, hypotension, acidosis, and hyperventilation are the most critical elements of anesthetic management.

8. Postoperative management

8.1. Postoperative management

The FHR and uterine activity should be monitored during recovery from anesthesia. Adequate analgesia should be obtained with systemic or spinal opioids. Prophylaxis against venous thrombosis should be considered.

Case study:

• Pregnant woman 30 weeks of pregnancy, she was complained from multiple menegiomas, conservative treatment was used throughout pregnancy period. This patient developed sever continuous vomiting, and rapid deterioration of nutritional status, neuro surgery team decided urgent operation for decompression of the brain, the patient was referred for obstetric, and anesthesia consultant.

• Anesthesia examination revealed that: Patient 35 years old 65 Kg, this the first baby, she complained from infertility for 15 years, she was hypertensive 150/90 on aldomit. Anticonvulsant drugs was administered, liver enzymes was 2

Folds, albumen was 2, 5, prothrombin was 65% kidney function within normal range. Hb was 6,5gm/dl, Obstetric examination revealed that baby nearly mature, his weight is under weight.

• Preoperative preparation:

Anesthesia consultant recommended blood transfusion for 4 units of packed RBCs, 4 units of human albumen, 4 units of fresh plasma 2 days before surgery. Preparations of another for units of fresh blood were for intraoperative losses Preoperative antacid was administered. Obstetric Preparations was for urgent cesarean section. Pediatric preparing to receive the premature neonate if urgent cesarean section was needed

• Anesthesia management:

• Monitoring:

Invasive blood pressure, ECG, end tidal CO2, pulse oximetry, uterine contraction monitor, fetal

Doppler. Positioning: Supine with left lateral tilt,

8.2. Induction of anesthesia

3-5 mg/kg sodium thiopental, Rocuronium 04 meg/kg, fentanyl 1mg/kg. Intubation by rapid sequence, the precautions mentioned above were considered

The operation was long 5 hours, blood loss was replaced, fetal heart was declined at third hour, urgent cesarean section was done, the pediatric consultant intubated the neonate, and he was incubated, for 2 weeks, he intubated and he is still living. Mother was in intensive care unit for 3 day

References

1. Heart Association. Coordinator of the series is Sidney C. Smith, Jr., M.D., Chief Science Officer, American Heart Association, Dallas, Tex. The series coordinator for *AFP* is Sumi Sexton, M.D.

2. Simon, R. H. Brain tumors in pregnancy. Semin Neurol (1988). , 8(3), 214-221.

3. Roelvink NCAKamphorst W, van Alphen HAM et al. Pregnancy-related primary brain and spinal tumors. Arch Neurol (1987). , 44, 209-215

4. (Schlehofer B, Blettner M, Wahrendorf J. Association between brain tumors and menopausal status. J Natl Cancer Inst 1992; 84 [17]: 1346-1349. 1983; 56: 974-977). 56, 974-977.

5. Harris, J. R, Morrow, M, & Bonadonna, G. Cancer of the breast. In DeVita VT, Hellman S, Rosenberg SA (eds). Cancer Principles and Practice of Oncology (Ed 4]. Philadelphia B Lippincott, (1993). , 1993, 1264-1332.

6. Roizen MF. Preoperative evaluation In: Miller RD, Eds.; Anesthesia. Vol. 1. Churchill. Livingstone New York, NY: 2000, p. 927-997

7. Malone DL, Genuit T, Tracy JK. Surgical site infections: reanalysis of risk factors. J Surg Res 2002; 103(1): 89-95.

8. Patel KL. Impact of tight glucose control on postoperative infection rates and wound healing in cardiac surgery patients. J Wound Ostomy Continence Nurs 2008; 35(4): 397-404

9. Cohn SL, Goldman L. Preoperative risk evaluation and perioperative management of patients with coronary artery disease. Med Clin North Am 2003; 87(1): 111-136

10. Chiu JW, White PF. Nonopioid intravenous anesthesia In: Barash PG, Cullen BF, Stoelting RK, Eds.; Clinical Anesthesia. 4th ed. Lippincott Williams and Wilkins Philadelphia, PA: 2001, p. 327-343

11. Landercasper J, Merz BJ, Cogbill TH. Perioperative stroke risk in 173 consecutive patients with a past history of stroke. Arch Surg 1990; 125: 986-989

12. Colson P, Ryckwaert F, Coriat P. Renin angiotensin system antagonists and anesthesia. Anesth Analg 1999; 89(5): 1143-1155

13. Bertrand M, Godet G, Meersschaert K. Should the angiotensin II antagonists be discontinued before surgery?. Anesth Analg 2001; 92(1): 26-30

14. Mercado DL, Petty BG. Perioperative medication management. Med Clin North Am 2003; 87: 41-57

15. Armstrong MJ, Schneck MJ, Biller J. Discontinuation of perioperative antiplatelet and anticoagulant therapy in stroke patients. Neurol Clin 2006; 24(4): 607-630

16. Traber KB. Preoperative evaluation In: Longnecker DE, Murphy FL, Eds.; Introduction to Anesthesia. 9th ed. WB Saunders Co Philadelphia, PA: 1997, p. 11-19

17. Brussel T, Chernow B. Perioperative management of endocrine problems: thyroid, adrenal cortex, pituitary. J Am Soc Anesthesiol 1990; 18: 33-48

18. Sarko J. Antidepressants, old and new: a review of their adverse effects and toxicity in overdose. Emerg Med Clin North Am 2000; 18: 637-654Goldberg JF. New drugs in psychiatry. Emerg Med Clin North Am 2000; 18(2): 211-231

19. Fleisher LA. Preoperative evaluation, In: Barash PG, Cullen BF, Stoelting RK, Eds.; Clinical Anesthesia. 4th ed. Lippincott Williams and Wilkins Philadelphia, PA: 2001, p. 473-489

20. Bradley PG, Menon DK. Preoperative evaluation of neurosurgical patients. Anaesth Intensive Care Med 2004; 5(10): 336-339

21. Practice Advisory for Preanesthesia Evaluation. A report by the American Society of Anesthesiologists Task Force on Preanesthesia evaluation. Anesthesiology 2002; 96: 485-496

22. Dempsey DT, Mullen JL, Buzby GP. The link between nutritional status and clinical outcome: can nutritional intervention modify it?. Am J Clin Nutr 1988; 47(S2): 352-356

23. Qaseem A, Snow V, Fitterman N. Risk assessment for and strategies to reduce perioperative pulmonary complications for patients undergoing non cardiothoracic surgery: a guideline from the American College of Physicians. Ann Intern Med 2006; 144(8): 575-580

24. Gibbs J, Cull W, Henderson W. Preoperative serum albumin level as a predictor of operative mortality and morbidity: results from the National VA Surgical Risk Study. Arch Surg 1999; 134(1): 36-42

25. Brown RDJr , Evans BA, Wiebers DO. Transient ischemic attack and minor ischemic stroke: an algorithm for evaluation and treatment. Mayo Clinic Division of Cerebrovascular Diseases. Mayo Clin Proc 1994; 69(11): 1027-1039

26. Joyce THIII. Prophylaxis for pulmonary acid aspiration. Am J Med 1987; 83(6A): 46-52

27. Fleisher LA, Beckman JA, Brown KA. ACC/AHA 2007 Guidelines on Perioperative Cardiovascular Evaluation and Care for Noncardiac Surgery: A Report of the American College of Cardiology/American Heart Association Task Force on Practice Guidelines (Writing Committee to Revise the 2002 Guidelines on Perioperative Cardiovascular Evaluation for Noncardiac Surgery) developed in collaboration with the American Society of Echocardiography, American Society of Nuclear Cardiology, Heart Rhythm Society, Society of Cardiovascular

Anesthesiologists, Society for Cardiovascular Angiography and Interventions, Society for Vascular Medicine and Biology, and Society for Vascular Surgery. J Am Coll Cardiol 2007; 50(17): e159-e241

28. Poldermans D, Boersma E, Bax JJ. Bisoprolol reduces cardiac death and myocardial infarction in high-risk patients as long as 2 years after successful major vascular surgery. Eur Heart J 2001; 22(15): 1353-1358

29. Mangano DT, Layug EL, Wallace A. Effect of atenolol on mortality and cardiovascular morbidity after noncardiac surgery. Multicenter Study of Perioperative Ischemia Research Group. N Engl J Med 1996; 335(23): 1713-1720

30. Hamilton MG, Hull RD, Pineo GF. Venous thromboembolism in neurosurgery and neurology: a review. Neurosurgery 1994; 34: 280-296

31. Lefevre F, Woolger JM. Surgery in the patient with neurologic disease. Med Clin North Am 2003; 87(1): 257-271

32. Meguid MM, Campos AC, Hammond WG. Nutritional support in surgical practice: Part II. Am J Surg 1990; 159(4): 427-443

33. Warner MA, Offord KP, Warner ME, Lennon RL, Conover MA, Jansson-Schumacher U. Role of preoperative cessation of smoking and other factors in postoperative pulmonary

complications: a blinded prospective study of coronary artery bypass patients. Mayo Clin Proc 1989; 64(6): 609-616

34. Larach MG, Rosenberg H, Gronert GA. Hyperkalemic cardiac arrest during anesthesia in infants and children with occult myopathies. Clin Pediatr (Phila) 1997; 36(1): 9-16

35. Kunst G, Graf BM, Schreiner R. Differential effects of sevoflurane, isoflurane, and halothane on Ca2+ release from the sarcoplasmic reticulum of skeletal muscle. Anesthesiology 1999; 91(1): 179-186

36. Birnkrant DJ, Panitch HB, Benditt JO. American College of Chest Physicians consensus statement on the respiratory and related management of patients with Duchenne muscular dystrophy undergoing anesthesia or sedation. Chest 2007; 132(6): 1977-1986

37. Baraka A. Anesthesia and myasthenia gravis. Can J Anaesth 1992; 39: 476-486

38. Seifert HS, Smith DS. Neuroanesthesia and neurologic disease In: Longnecker DE, Murphy FL, Eds.; Introduction to Anesthesia. 9th ed. WB Saunders Co Philadelphia, PA: 1997, p. 400-414

39. Dierdorf SF. Anesthesia for patients with rare and coexisting disease In: Barash PG, Cullen BF, Stoelting RK, Eds.; Clinical Anesthesia. 4th ed. Philadelphia, PA: 2001, p. 491-520

40. Turnbull JM, Buck C. The value of preoperative screening investigations in otherwise healthy individuals. Arch Intern Med 1987; 147(6): 1101-1105

41. Limburg M, Wijdicks EF, Li H. Ischemic stroke after surgical procedures: clinical features, neuroimaging, and risk factors. Neurology 1998; 50(4): 895-901

42. Restrepo L, Wityk RJ, Grega MA. Diffusion- and perfusion-weighted magnetic resonance imaging of the brain before and after coronary artery bypass grafting surgery. Stroke 2002; 33(12): 2909-2915

43. Kluger J, White CM. Amiodarone prevents symptomatic atrial fibrillation and reduces the risk of cerebrovascular accidents and ventricular tachycardia after open heart surgery: results of the Atrial Fibrillation Suppression Trial (AFIST). Card Electrophysiol Rev 2003; 7(2): 165-167

44. Haas, J. F, Janisch, W, & Staneczek, W. Newly diagnosed primary intracranial neoplasms in pregnant women: a population-based assessment. J Neurol Neurosurg Psychiatry (1986). , 49, 874-880.

45. Cifuentes, N, & Pickren, J. W. Metastases from carcinoma of mammary gland: an autopsy study. J Surg Oncol (1979). , 11, 193-205.

46. Anderson, N. E. Neurological complications of breast cancer. In Wiley RG (ed). Neurological Complications of Cancer. New York: Marcel Dekker, (1995). , 1995, 311-332.

47. Hall, S. M, Buzdar, A. U, & Blumenschein, G. R. Cranial nerve palsies in metastatic breast cancer due to osseous metastasis without intracranial involvement. Cancer (1983). , 52, 180-184.

48. Greenberg, H, Deck, M, & Vikram, B. Metastasis to the base of the skull: clinical findings in 43 patients. Neurology (1981). , 31, 530-537.

49. Doll, D. C, Ringenberg, S, & Yarbro, J. W. Management of cancer during pregnancy.Arch Intern Med (1988). , 148, 2058-2064.

50. Glick, R. P, Penny, D, & Hart, A. The pre-operative and post-operative management of the brain tumor patient. In Morantz RA, Walsh JW (eds). Brain Tumors. New York: Marcel Dekker, (1994). , 1994, 345-366.

51. Carpenter, T. M. Murlin JR: The energy metabolism of mother and child just before and just after birth. *AMA Arch Intern Med* (1911). , 7, 184-222.

52. Root, H. Root HK: The basal metabolism during pregnancy and the puerperium. *ArchIntern Med* (1923). , 32, 411-424.

53. Sandiford, I, & Wheeler, T. The basal metabolism before, during, and after pregnancyJ Bio Chem. lxii: 329-52.

54. Caton, D, Henderson, D. J, & Wilcox, C. J. Barron DH: *Oxygen consumption of the uterus and its contents and*

weight at birth of lambs. In: Longo LD, Reneau DD, ed. Fetal and

55. Newborn Cardiovascular Physiology, 2. New York: Garland STPM Press; (1978). vv28.,1978, 123-134.

56. Yankowitz, J. *Use of medications in pregnancy: General principles, teratology, and current developments*. In: Yankowitz J, Niebyl JR, ed. *Drug Therapy in Pregnancy*, Baltimore: Lippincott Williams & Wilkins; (2001).

57. Bain, M. D, Copas, D. K, & Landon, M. J l. In vivo permeability of the human placenta to inulin and mannitol. J Physiol (1988). , 399, 313-319.

58. Basso, A, Fernandez, A, Althabe, O, et al. Passage of mannitol from mother to amniotic fluid and fetus. Obstet Gynecol (1977). , 49(5), 628-631.

59. Evaluation of the Pregnant Patient *Robert Gaiser MD* ANESTHESIOLOGY Edited By:David E. Longnecker, MD, FRCARobert D. Dripps David L. Brown, MD Mark F.Newman, MD,Warren M. Zapol, MD Copyright © (2008). by The McGraw-Hill Companies,Inc.. CHAPTER 21 358

60. Buehler, B. A, Delimont, D, & Van Waes, M. Finnell RH: Prenatal prediction of risk of the fetal hydantoin syndrome. N Engl J Med (1990). , 322, 1567-1572.

61. Teratology Society Public Affairs Committee FDA classification of drugs for teratogenic risk. Teratology (1994). , 49, 446-447.

62. Friedman JM: Report of the Teratology Society Public Affairs Committee Symposium on FDA Classification of Drugs Teratology (1993). , 48, 5-6.

63. Doering, P. L, Boothby, L. A, & Cheok, M. Review of pregnancy labeling of prescription drugs: Is the current system adequate to inform of risks?. Am J Obstet Gynecol (2002). ,187, 333-339.

64. Malone, F. D, & Alton, D. ME: Drugs in pregnancy: Anticonvulsants. *Semin Perinatol* (1997). , 21, 114-123.

65. Morrell MJ: Guidelines for the care of women with epilepsy *Neurology* (1998). Suppl 4):SS 27., 21.

66. Shapiro, S, Hartz, S. C, Siskind, V, et al. Anticonvulsants and parental epilepsy in the development of birth defects. Lancet (1976). i:, 272-275.

67. Holmes, L. B, Rosenberger, P. B, Harvey, E. A, et al. Intelligence and physical features of children of women with epilepsy. *Teratology* (2000). , 61, 196-202.

68. Holmes, L. B, Harvey, E. A, Cull, B. A, et al. The teratogenicity of anticonvulsant drugs.*N Engl J Med* (2001). , 344, 1132-1138.

69. American College of Obstetricians and Gynecologists Teratology. ACOG Educational Bulletin April (1997). (236)

70. Sever, L. E. Mortensen ME: *Teratology and the epidemiology of birth defects: Occupational and environmental perspectives.* In: Gabbe SG, Niebyl JR, Simpson JL, ed. *Obstetrics: Normal and Problem*

Pregnancies, 3rd edition. New York: Churchill Livingston; (1996).

71. American College of Obstetricians and Gynecologists Assessment of risk factors for preterm birth. ACOG Practice Bulletin October (2001). Liver to perinatal mortality. Br Med J 1976; 2(31), 965-968.

72. Villar, J, Ezcurra, E. J, De La Fuente, V. G, & Canpodonico, L. Pre-term delivery syndrome, the unmet need. Res Clin Forums (1994). , 16, 9-33.

73. Tucker, J. M, Goldenberg, R. L, Davis, R. O, et al. Etiologies of preterm birth in an indigent population: is prevention a logical expectation? Obstet Gynecol (1991). , 77,343-347.

74. Curtin, S. C. Recent changes in birth attendant, place of birth, and the use of obstetric interventions: United States, J Nurse Midwifery (1999). , 1989-1997.

75. Goodlin, R. C. History of fetal monitoring. Am J Obstet Gynecol (1979).

76. [36] Kelso, I. M, Parsons, R. J, Lawrence, G. F, et al. An assessment of continuous fetal heart rate monitoring in labor: a randomized trial. Am J Obstet Gynecol (1978)

77. Reuwer, P. J, Bruinse, H. W, & Stoutenbeek, T. Doppler assessment of the fetoplacental circulation in normal and growth-retarded fetuses. Eur J Obstet Gynecol Reprod Biol (1984).

78. Vintzileos, A. M, Nioka, S, Lake, M, et al. Transabdominal fetal pulse oximetry with near-infrared spectroscopy. Am J Obstet Gynecol (2005).

79. Martin, J. A, Hamilton, B. E, Sutton, P. D, et al. Births: Final Data for 2002; National Vital Statistics Reports, Hyattsville, MD: National Center for Health Statistics, (2003). ,52(10)

80. Hack, M, & Fanaroff, A. A. Outcomes of extremely immature infants: a perinatal dilemmN Engl J Med (1993).

81. Mccormick, M. C. The contribution of low birth weight to infant mortality and childhood morbidity. N Engl J Med (1985).

82. Bradić Z[1], Ivanović B, Marković D, Simić D, Janković R, Kalezić N. **Preoperative preparation of patients with cardiomyopathies in non-cardiac surgery.**

83. **Acta Chir Iugosl.** 2011;58(2):39-43.

84. Eagle KA, Berger PB, Calkins H, Chaitman BR, Ewy GA, Fleischmann KE, et al. ACC/AHA guideline update for perioperative cardiovascular evaluation for noncardiac surgery—executive summary: a report of the American College of Cardiology/American Heart Association Task Force on Practice Guidelines (Committee to Update the 1996 Guidelines on Perioperative Cardiovascular Evaluation for Noncardiac Surgery). *J Am Coll Cardiol.* 2002; 39:542–53.

85. Morris CK, Ueshima K, Kawaguchi T, Hideg A, Froelicher VF. The prognostic value of exercise capacity: a review of the literature. *Am Heart J*. 1991; 122:1423–31.

86. Reilly DF, McNeely MJ, Doerner D, Greenberg DL, Staiger TO, Geist MJ, et al. Self-reported exercise tolerance and the risk of serious perioperative complications. *Arch Intern Med*. 1999;159:2185–92.

87. Fleisher LA. Cardiac risk in noncardiac surgery: new insights in management. *ACC Curr J Rev*. 2005; 14:5–8.

88. McFalls EO, Ward HB, Moritz TE, Goldman S, Krupski WC, Littooy F, et al. Coronary-artery revascularization before elective major vascular surgery. *N Engl J Med*. 2004;351:2795–804.

89. Kaluza GL, Joseph J, Lee JR, Raizner ME, Raizner AE. Catastrophic outcomes of noncardiac surgery soon after coronary stenting. *J Am Coll Cardiol*. 2000; 35:1288–94.

90. Wilson SH, Fasseas P, Orford JL, Lennon RJ, Horlocker T, Charnoff NE, et al. Clinical outcome of patients undergoing non-cardiac surgery in the two months following coronary stenting. *J Am Coll Cardiol*. 2003; 42:234–40.

91. Goldman L, Caldera DL, Nussbaum SR, Southwick FS, Krogstad D, Murray B, et al. Multifactorial index of cardiac risk in noncardiac surgical procedures. *N Engl J Med*. 1977; 297:845–50.

92. Detsky AS, Abrams HB, For bath N, Scott JG, Hilliard JR. Cardiac assessment for patients undergoing noncardiac

surgery. A multifactorial clinical risk index. *Arch Intern Med.* 1986; 146:2131–4.

93. Lee TH, Marc Antonio ER, Mangione CM, Thomas EJ, Polanczyk CA, Cook EF, et al. Derivation and prospective validation of a simple index for prediction of cardiac risk of major noncardiac surgery. *Circulation.* 1999;100:1043–9.

94. Mangano DT, Layug EL, Wallace A, Tateo I. Effect of atenolol on mortality and cardiovascular morbidity after noncardiac surgery. Multicenter Study of Perioperative Ischemia Research Group [Published correction appears in N Engl J Med 1997; 336:1039]. *N Engl J Med.* 1996; 335:1713–20.

95. Poldermans D, Boersma E, Bax JJ, Thomson IR, van de Ven LL, Blankensteijn JD, et al. The effect of bisoprolol on perioperative mortality and myocardial infarction in high-risk patients undergoing vascular surgery. Dutch Echocardiographic Cardiac Risk Evaluation Applying Stress Echocardiography Study Group. *N Engl J Med.* 1999; 341:1789–94.

96. Brady AR, Gibbs JS, Greenhalgh RM, Powell JT, Sydes MR. Perioperative beta-blockade (POBBLE) for patients undergoing infrarenal vascular surgery: results of a randomized double-blind controlled trial. *J Vasc Surg.* 2005; 41:602–9.

97. Stone JG, Foex P, Sear JW, Johnson LL, Khambatta HJ, Triner L. Myocardial ischemia in untreated hypertensive patients: effect of a single small oral dose of a beta-

adrenergic blocking agent. *Anesthesiology*. 1988; 68:495–500.

98. Raby KE, Brull SJ, Timimi F, Akhtar S, Rosenbaum S, Naimi C, et al. The effect of heart rate control on myocardial ischemia among high-risk patients after vascular surgery. *Anesth Analg*. 1999; 88:477–82.

99. Wallace A, Layug B, Tateo I, Li J, Hollenberg M, Browner W, et al. Prophylactic atenolol reduces postoperative myocardial ischemia. McSPI Research Group. *Anesthesiology*. 1998; 88:7–17.

100. Zaugg M, Tagliente T, Lucchinetti E, Jacobs E, Krol M, Bodian C, et al. Beneficial effects from beta-adrenergic blockade in elderly patients undergoing noncardiac surgery. *Anesthesiology*. 1999; 91:1674–86.

101. Urban MK, Markowitz SM, Gordon MA, Urquhart BL, Kligfield P. Postoperative prophylactic administration of beta-adrenergic blockers in patients at risk for myocardial ischemia. *Anesth Analg*. 2000; 90:1257–61.

102. Juul AB, Wetterslev J, Gluud C, Kofoed-Enevoldsen A, Jensen G, Callesen T, et al., for the DIPOM Trial Group. Effect of perioperative beta blockade in patients with diabetes undergoing major non-cardiac surgery: randomised placebo controlled, blinded multicentre trial. *BMJ*. 2006; 332:1482.

103. Lindenauer PK, Pekow P, Wang K, Mamidi DK, Gutierrez B, Benjamin EM. Perioperative beta-blocker

therapy and mortality after major non-cardiac surgery. *N Engl J Med*. 2005; 353:349–61.

104.   Devereaux PJ, Beattie WS, Choi PT, Badner NH, Guyatt GH, Villar JC, et al. How strong is the evidence for the use of perioperative beta blockers in non-cardiac surgery? Systematic review and meta-analysis of randomised controlled trials. *BMJ*. 2005; 331:313–21.

105.   Fringe HH, Bax JJ, Boersma E, Kertai MD, Meij SH, Galal W, et al. High-dose beta-blockers and tight heart rate control reduce myocardial ischemia and troponin T release in vascular surgery patients. *Circulation*. 2006; 114(1 suppl) I344–9.

106.   Fleisher LA, Beckman JA, Brown KA, Calkins H, Chaikof E, Fleischmann KE, et al. ACC/AHA 2006 guideline update on perioperative cardiovascular evaluation for noncardiac surgery: focused update on perioperative beta-blocker therapy: a report of the American College of Cardiology/American Heart Association Task Force on Practice Guidelines (Writing Committee to Update the 2002 Guidelines on Perioperative Cardiovascular Evaluation for Noncardiac Surgery) developed in collaboration with the American Society of Echocardiography, American Society of Nuclear Cardiology, Heart Rhythm Society, Society of Cardiovascular Anesthesiologists, Society for Cardiovascular Angiography and Interventions, and Society for Vascular Medicine and Biology. *J Am Coll Cardiol*. 2006; 47:2343–55.

107.   Redelmeier D, Scales D, Kopp A. Beta blockers for elective surgery in elderly patients: population based, retrospective cohort study. *BMJ*. 2005; 331:932.

108.   Stamler JS, Loh E, Roddy MA, Currie KE, Creager MA. Nitric oxide regulates basal systemic and pulmonary vascular resistance in healthy humans. *Circulation*. 1994;89:2035–40.

109.   Kurowska EM. Nitric oxide therapies in vascular diseases. *Curr Pharm Des*. 2002; 8:155–66.

110.   Carrasco LR, Chou JC. Perioperative management of patients with renal disease. ORAL MAXILLOFAC SURG CLIN NORTH AM. 2006 May. 18(2):203-12, VI. [Medline].

111.   Xu GG, Yam A, Teoh LC, Yong FC, Tay SC. Epidemiology and management of surgical upper limb infections in patients with end-stage renal failure. ANN ACAD MED SINGAPORE. 2010 Sep. 39(9):670-5.[Medline].

112.   Bauer LA, Black D, Gensler A. Procainamide-cimetidine drug interaction in elderly male patients. J AM GERIATR SOC. 1990 Apr. 38(4):467-9. [Medline].

113.   Eagle KA, Berger PB, Calkins H, Chaitman BR, Ewy GA, Fleischmann KE, et al. ACC/AHA guideline update for perioperative cardiovascular evaluation for noncardiac surgery--executive summary: a report of the American College of Cardiology/American Heart Association Task

Force on Practice Guidelines (Committee to Update the 1996 Guidelines on Perioperative Cardiovascular Evaluation for Noncardiac Surgery). J AM COLL CARDIOL. 2002 Feb 6. 39(3):542-53. [Medline].

114.   [Guideline] Fleisher LA, Fleischmann KE, Auerbach AD, Barnason SA, Beckman JA, Bozkurt B, et al. 2014 ACC/AHA guideline on perioperative cardiovascular evaluation and management of patients undergoing noncardiac surgery: executive summary: a report of the American College of Cardiology/American Heart Association Task Force on Practice Guidelines. CIRCULATION. 2014 Dec 9. 130 (24):2215-45. [Medline]. [Full Text].

115.   [Guideline] Washam JB, Herzog CA, Beitelshees AL, et al. Pharmacotherapy in chronic kidney disease patients presenting with acute coronary syndrome: a scientific statement from the American Heart Association. CIRCULATION. 2015 Mar 24. 131 (12):1123-49. [Medline]. [Full Text].

116.   Baglin A, Hanslik T, Vaillant JN, Boulard JC, Moulonguet-Doleris L, Prinseau J. Severe valvular heart disease in patients on chronic dialysis. A five-year multicenter French survey. ANN MED INTERN

117.   van Haelst PL, van Doormaal JJ, May JF, Gans RO, Crijns HJ, Cohen Tervaert JW. Secondary prevention with fluvastatin decreases levels of adhesion molecules, neopterin and C-reactive protein. *Eur J Intern Med.* 2001; 12:503–9.

118.   Kertai MD, Boersma E, Westerhout CM, Klein J, Van Urk H, Bax JJ, et al. A combination of statins and beta-blockers is independently associated with a reduction in the incidence of perioperative mortality and nonfatal myocardial infarction in patients undergoing abdominal aortic aneurysm surgery. *Eur J Vasc Endovasc Surg.* 2004; 28:343–52.

119.   Poldermans D, Bax JJ, Kertai MD, Krenning B, Westerhout CM, Schinkel AF, et al. Statins are associated with a reduced incidence of perioperative mortality in patients undergoing major noncardiac vascular surgery. *Circulation.* 2003; 107:1848–51.

120.   O'Neil-Callahan K, Katsimaglis G, Tepper MR, Ryan J, Mosby C, Ioannidis JP, et al. Statins decrease perioperative cardiac complications in patients undergoing noncardiac vascular surgery: the Statins for Risk Reduction in Surgery (StaRRS) study. *J Am Coll Cardiol.* 2005; 45:336–42.

121.   Durazzo AE, Machado FS, Ikeoka DT, De Bernoche C, Monachini MC, Puech-Leao P, et al. Reduction in cardiovascular events after vascular surgery with atorvastatin: a randomized trial. *J Vasc Surg.* 2004; 39:967–75.

122.   Lindenauer PK, Pekow P, Wang K, Gutierrez B, Benjamin EM. Lipid-lowering therapy and in-hospital

mortality following major noncardiac surgery. *JAMA*. 2004; 291:2092–9.

123.   Stuhmeier KD, Mainzer B, Cierpka J, Sandmann W, Tarnow J. Small, oral dose of clonidine reduces the incidence of intraoperative myocardial ischemia in patients having vascular surgery.*Anesthesiology*. 1996;85:706–12.

124.   Wijeysundera DN, Naik JS, Beattie WS. Alpha-2 adrenergic agonists to prevent perioperative cardiovascular complications: a meta-analysis. *Am J Med*. 2003;114:742–52.

125.   Stevens RD, Burri H, Tramer MR. Pharmacologic myocardial protection in patients undergoing noncardiac surgery: a quantitative systematic review. *Anesth Analg*. 2003; 97:623–33.

126.   Nishina K, Mikawa K, Uesugi T, Obara H, Maekawa M, Kamae I, et al. Efficacy of clonidine for prevention of perioperative myocardial ischemia: a critical appraisal and meta-analysis of the literature. *Anesthesiology*. 2002;96:323–9.

127.   Wallace AW, Galindez D, Salahieh A, Layug EL, Lazo EA, Haratonik KA, et al. Effect of clonidine on cardiovascular morbidity and mortality after noncardiac surgery. *Anesthesiology*. 2004; 101:284–93.

128.   Ellis JE, Drijvers G, Pedlow S, Laff SP, Sorrentino MJ, Foss JF, et al. Pre-medication with oral and transdermal clonidine provides safe and efficacious postoperative sympatholysis. *Anesth Analg*. 1994;79:1133–40.

129.   Perioperative sympatholysis. Beneficial effects of the alpha 2-adre-noceptor agonist mivazerol on hemodynamic stability and myocardial ischemia. McSPI—Europe Research Group.*Anesthesiology*. 1997; 86:346–63.

130.   Sear JW, Higham H. Issues in the perioperative management of the elderly patient with cardiovascular disease. *Drugs Aging*. 2002; 19:429–51.

131.   Kakisis JD, Abir F, Liapis CD, Sumpio BE. An appraisal of different cardiac risk reduction strategies in vascular surgery patients. *Eur J Vasc Endovasc Surg*. 2003; 25:493–504.